Parvovirus B19: How to Avoid it, and its Potential Impact

1. Introduction to Parvovirus (Slapped Cheek Disease)

Parvovirus B19 is a small, non-enveloped DNA virus that belongs to the Parvoviridae family.

This virus is the causative agent of several clinical conditions, the most common of which is erythema infectiosum, also known as "slapped cheek disease" due to the characteristic facial rash it causes.

First identified in the 1970s, Parvovirus B19 is widely recognized for its role in childhood infections, though it can affect individuals of all ages.

The virus is particularly notable for its ability to infect only humans, making it distinct from other parvoviruses that can infect animals.

Parvovirus B19 targets the erythroid progenitor cells in the bone marrow, which are crucial for the production of red blood cells.

As a result, the virus can lead to a transient halt in red blood cell production, especially in individuals with underlying health conditions, leading to various clinical manifestations.

History and Naming of "Slapped Cheek Disease"

The term "slapped cheek disease" originates from one of the most recognizable symptoms of the infection: a bright red rash that appears on the face, resembling the impression of a slap.

This rash is often accompanied by a lace-like rash on the trunk and limbs, further distinguishing it from other viral rashes.

Erythema infectiosum, the
medical term for the condition,
is considered one of the classic
childhood exanthems, along
with measles, rubella,
chickenpox, and roseola.

Historically, these diseases
were among the most common
causes of rashes and fevers in
children, often spreading rapidly
through communities due to
their highly contagious nature.

The recognition of erythema infectiosum as a distinct clinical entity dates back to the early 20th century, but it wasn't until the identification of Parvovirus B19 that the specific cause of the disease was understood.

The discovery of the virus was a significant milestone in virology and has since led to a better understanding of the disease and its management.

Symptoms and Signs

The clinical presentation of Parvovirus B19 infection can vary depending on the age and immune status of the individual.

However, several hallmark symptoms are commonly associated with "slapped cheek disease."

- Facial Rash: The most distinctive feature is the bright red rash on the cheeks, which gives the appearance of a slapped face. This rash is typically symmetrical and may extend to the forehead and chin.

- Lacy Rash on the Body: After the facial rash, a second rash often appears on the trunk and limbs. This rash has a reticular or lace-like pattern and can be mildly itchy. The body rash may come and go, often triggered by factors like heat, sunlight, or stress.

- Fever: A mild fever often precedes the appearance of the rash by a few days. The fever is generally low-grade and may be accompanied by other nonspecific symptoms such as malaise, headache, and muscle aches.

- Joint Pain: In some cases, particularly in older children and adults, the infection may cause joint pain and swelling. This symptom is more common in women and can mimic conditions like rheumatoid arthritis.

- Respiratory Symptoms: Some individuals may experience mild respiratory symptoms, including a sore throat, runny nose, and cough, particularly in the early stages of infection.

The rash and joint symptoms are thought to be immune-mediated, resulting from the body's response to the virus rather than direct viral damage. The symptoms typically resolve on their own within a few weeks, although joint pain can persist for longer in some cases.

Demographics: Who is Most at Risk?

Parvovirus B19 is a ubiquitous virus, meaning it is found worldwide and can infect individuals of all ages.

However, certain groups are more susceptible to infection and its complications:

- Children: The primary age group affected by erythema infectiosum is school-aged children, typically between 5 and 15 years old. The virus spreads easily in settings where children are in close contact, such as schools and daycare centers.

- Pregnant Women: Pregnant women are at risk of passing the virus to their fetus if they become infected, especially during the first and second trimesters. This can lead to severe complications, including fetal anemia, hydrops fetalis, and even miscarriage.

- Immunocompromised Individuals: Those with weakened immune systems, such as individuals undergoing chemotherapy, organ transplant recipients, or those with HIV/AIDS, are at higher risk for severe or prolonged infection.

 These individuals may develop chronic anemia due to the virus's impact on red blood cell production.

- Individuals with Hematological Disorders: People with conditions like sickle cell disease or hereditary spherocytosis, which affect red blood cell production or lifespan, are particularly vulnerable. In these cases, Parvovirus B19 can cause an aplastic crisis, a sudden and severe drop in red blood cells.

Understanding these risk factors is crucial for implementing preventive measures and for the early identification of cases that may require more intensive management.

Transmission and Contagiousness

Parvovirus B19 is highly contagious, primarily spreading through respiratory secretions, such as saliva, sputum, or nasal mucus, particularly when an infected person coughs or sneezes.

The virus can also spread through blood transfusions or from a pregnant woman to her fetus.

The contagious period typically occurs before the onset of the rash, during which time the virus is actively replicating and shedding.

Once the rash appears, the risk of transmission significantly decreases, as the virus is no longer present in the respiratory secretions.

The virus is resilient in the environment, capable of surviving on surfaces for several days, which facilitates its spread in community settings like schools.

Due to its mode of transmission, close contact with an infected individual, such as sharing eating utensils or being in crowded, enclosed spaces, increases the risk of infection.

In summary, Parvovirus B19 is a common, highly contagious virus that primarily affects children but can have serious consequences in certain populations.

Understanding its transmission, symptoms, and risk factors is essential for managing and preventing outbreaks, particularly in school settings where the virus can spread rapidly.

2. Understanding the Impact of Parvovirus

In children, Parvovirus B19 is usually a mild illness, but it can lead to significant discomfort and, in rare cases, complications.

The primary concern with Parvovirus in children is its ability to cause outbreaks in schools, where it spreads quickly among susceptible individuals.

- Symptoms: In children, the disease typically begins with nonspecific symptoms such as a low-grade fever, fatigue, and a runny nose, which are often mistaken for a common cold.

 After a few days, the characteristic facial rash develops, followed by the lacy rash on the body. The illness is usually self-limiting, and most children recover fully within a couple of weeks.

- Complications: Although rare, complications can occur, particularly in children with underlying conditions like chronic hemolytic anemia.

 These children are at risk of developing an aplastic crisis, where the bone marrow temporarily stops producing red blood cells, leading to severe anemia. This condition requires immediate medical attention and may necessitate a blood transfusion.

- Impact on School Attendance: The contagious nature of the virus and the prolonged rash phase, during which children may not feel well enough to attend school, can result in significant absenteeism.

 This, in turn, can disrupt learning and place additional burdens on families and educators.

Parvovirus in Pregnant Women

Parvovirus B19 poses a significant risk to pregnant women, particularly during the first half of pregnancy.

The virus can cross the placenta and infect the fetus, potentially leading to severe outcomes.

- Fetal Risks: The most concerning complication of Parvovirus infection during pregnancy is hydrops fetalis, a condition where the fetus develops severe anemia, leading to heart failure and fluid accumulation in the body.

 In some cases, this can result in fetal death. The risk of these complications is highest if the mother is infected between the 9th and 20th weeks of pregnancy.

- Maternal Symptoms: Pregnant women may experience the typical symptoms of erythema infectiosum, including the rash and joint pain.

 However, they may also have more severe or prolonged symptoms, and the psychological stress of knowing the potential risks to the fetus can be significant.

- Management: Pregnant women who are exposed to Parvovirus or develop symptoms should seek medical attention promptly.

 Ultrasounds may be used to monitor the fetus for signs of anemia or hydrops, and in severe cases, intrauterine blood transfusions may be necessary to save the fetus.

Parvovirus in Immunocompromised Individuals

 For individuals with compromised immune systems, Parvovirus B19 can cause chronic or severe disease due to the body's inability to clear the virus effectively.

- Chronic Infection: In immunocompromised patients, the virus may persist in the body, leading to chronic anemia. This can result in ongoing symptoms such as fatigue, pallor, and shortness of breath.

  Managing these cases often requires specialized care, including immunoglobulin therapy to help the body fight the virus.

- Increased Risk of Complications: These individuals are also at higher risk for complications such as myocarditis (inflammation of the heart muscle) or encephalitis (inflammation of the brain), although these are rare.

- Preventive Measures: Immunocompromised individuals, including those undergoing chemotherapy or living with HIV/AIDS, should take extra precautions to avoid exposure to Parvovirus, particularly during outbreaks in the community.

Short-term and Long-term Complications

 While most cases of Parvovirus B19 infection resolve without lasting effects, there are potential short-term and long-term complications that can arise, particularly in vulnerable populations.

- Short-term Complications:
These include severe anemia in
individuals with pre-existing
blood disorders, joint pain that
can mimic arthritis, and in some
cases, myocarditis or
encephalitis.

 In children, the illness can lead
to significant absenteeism from
school and may require medical
intervention for complications.

- Long-term Complications: Chronic anemia is the most significant long-term complication, particularly in immunocompromised patients.

 There have also been reports of chronic arthritis following infection, particularly in adults. In pregnant women, the long-term impact may include the psychological effects of dealing with a complicated pregnancy or fetal loss.

Understanding the potential complications of Parvovirus B19 infection is crucial for managing the disease and providing appropriate care to those affected.

3. How to Avoid Parvovirus Infection

Preventive Measures in Schools and Daycare Centers

Schools and daycare centers are common settings for the spread of Parvovirus B19 due to the close contact among children and staff.

Implementing preventive measures can significantly reduce the risk of an outbreak.

- Regular Handwashing:

 Encouraging frequent handwashing with soap and water among students and staff is one of the most effective ways to prevent the spread of Parvovirus.

 Schools should ensure that handwashing facilities are easily accessible and well-stocked with supplies.

- Surface Cleaning: Regular cleaning and disinfection of surfaces, particularly those frequently touched like doorknobs, desks, and toys, can help minimize the spread of the virus.

  Schools should establish a routine cleaning schedule and ensure that all areas are properly sanitized.

- Educating Staff and Students: Providing education about the signs and symptoms of Parvovirus B19, as well as the importance of staying home when sick, can help reduce transmission.

 Schools should distribute informational materials and hold briefings for staff and parents to keep everyone informed.

- Isolating Infected Individuals: Children or staff members who develop symptoms of Parvovirus B19 should be sent home and advised to avoid contact with others until they are no longer contagious.

 This is particularly important during the early stages of the illness, when the virus is most likely to spread.

- Ventilation: Improving ventilation in classrooms and common areas can reduce the concentration of airborne viruses, including Parvovirus B19.

 Schools should ensure that ventilation systems are functioning properly and consider opening windows to increase air circulation when weather permits.

Personal Hygiene Practices

Personal hygiene is a key component of preventing the spread of Parvovirus B19.

Both children and adults should be encouraged to adopt the following practices:

- Hand Hygiene: Washing hands frequently with soap and water, especially after coughing, sneezing, or touching the face, can help prevent the spread of the virus.

 If soap and water are not available, using an alcohol-based hand sanitizer is a good alternative.

- Respiratory Etiquette:
Covering the mouth and nose
with a tissue or elbow when
coughing or sneezing can reduce
the spread of respiratory
droplets that carry the virus.

 Used tissues should be disposed
of immediately, and hands
should be washed afterward.

- Avoiding Close Contact: Individuals who are sick should avoid close contact with others, especially those who are vulnerable to severe disease, such as pregnant women, immunocompromised individuals, and those with chronic health conditions.

- Avoiding Sharing Personal Items: Sharing items such as drinking glasses, eating utensils, and towels should be avoided, as these can be vehicles for spreading the virus.

Role of Vaccinations and Immunity

Currently, there is no vaccine available for Parvovirus B19, which makes prevention through other means even more critical.

However, understanding immunity can help manage the risk of infection.

- Natural Immunity: After a person is infected with Parvovirus B19, they typically develop immunity, which usually lasts for life.

 This means that individuals who have had the virus before are unlikely to be reinfected.

 However, because many adults have been exposed to the virus as children, a significant portion of the population is already immune.

- Population Immunity: High levels of immunity in a population can help reduce the spread of the virus, as fewer people are susceptible to infection.

 This is particularly important in preventing outbreaks in schools and other community settings.

- Monitoring Immunity: In certain high-risk situations, such as in healthcare settings or among pregnant women, it may be advisable to test for immunity to Parvovirus B19, particularly if there is known exposure or an ongoing outbreak.

Community Health Measures

 Beyond individual and school-based prevention efforts, community-wide measures are essential for controlling the spread of Parvovirus B19.

- Surveillance and Reporting: Public health authorities should conduct surveillance to monitor the incidence of Parvovirus B19 and detect outbreaks early.

 Schools and healthcare providers play a critical role in reporting cases to public health officials.

- Public Awareness Campaigns: Educating the public about Parvovirus B19, its symptoms, and how it spreads can help individuals take proactive steps to protect themselves and others.

 Public health campaigns should focus on high-risk groups and settings where the virus is most likely to spread.

- Outbreak Management: In the event of an outbreak, public health officials should implement measures to limit the spread of the virus.

 This may include recommending temporary school closures, advising against large gatherings, and providing guidance on hygiene practices.

Managing Outbreaks: Protocols and Procedures

When an outbreak of Parvovirus B19 occurs, swift action is necessary to prevent widespread transmission.

Schools and public health authorities should have protocols in place to manage such situations.

- Case Identification and Isolation: Early identification of cases is critical.

 Once a case is confirmed, the affected individual should be isolated from others to prevent further spread.

 Schools should have clear guidelines on how to handle symptomatic students and staff.

- Communication with Parents and Staff: Transparent and timely communication is essential during an outbreak.

 Schools should inform parents and staff about the situation, what steps are being taken, and what they can do to protect themselves and their families.

- Collaboration with Health Authorities: Schools should work closely with local health departments to manage outbreaks. This includes sharing information about cases, implementing recommended control measures, and following public health guidance.

- Contingency Planning: Schools should have contingency plans in place for dealing with significant outbreaks, including options for remote learning, adjusting schedules, and providing support to affected families.

Implementing these preventive measures can significantly reduce the risk of Parvovirus B19 spreading in schools and the broader community, protecting vulnerable individuals and minimizing disruptions to education.

4. Impact on the New School Year

Potential Risks of an Outbreak in Schools

As schools reopen for the new academic year, the risk of Parvovirus B19 outbreaks is a genuine concern, particularly in areas where the virus is known to circulate.

Several factors could increase the likelihood of an outbreak:

- High Density of Students: Schools are environments where students spend extended periods in close proximity, making it easy for the virus to spread through respiratory droplets and contact with contaminated surfaces.

- Increased Social Interaction: The beginning of the school year often involves increased social interaction as students, teachers, and staff return from summer breaks. This can facilitate the spread of the virus, especially if some individuals are asymptomatic carriers.

- Lack of Immunity in Younger Students: Younger students, particularly those in preschool or early elementary school, may not have been previously exposed to Parvovirus B19 and, therefore, lack immunity.

 This makes them more susceptible to infection and can lead to higher rates of transmission within this age group.

- Challenges in Enforcing Hygiene Practices: Ensuring that young children consistently follow hygiene practices, such as handwashing and avoiding face touching, can be difficult, increasing the risk of transmission.

- Potential for Misdiagnosis: The early symptoms of Parvovirus B19, such as mild fever and cold-like symptoms, can be easily mistaken for other common illnesses, leading to delays in diagnosis and increased risk of spread within the school.

How Schools Can Prepare for Parvovirus

Preparation is key to minimizing the impact of a Parvovirus B19 outbreak on the school community.

Schools can take several proactive steps to be ready for the new school year:

- Developing a Response Plan: Schools should have a clear plan in place for responding to a Parvovirus B19 outbreak.

 This plan should outline procedures for identifying and isolating cases, communicating with parents and staff, and working with health authorities.

- Training Staff: Teachers, administrators, and school health personnel should receive training on how to recognize the symptoms of Parvovirus B19, implement hygiene protocols, and handle potential cases.

 This training should also include guidelines on when to send students home and how to support affected families.

- Promoting Vaccinations:

 While there is no vaccine for Parvovirus B19, promoting vaccinations against other common illnesses can help reduce the overall burden of illness in schools and make it easier to identify and manage Parvovirus cases when they occur.

- Enhanced Cleaning Protocols:

  Schools should implement enhanced cleaning protocols, particularly in high-touch areas like classrooms, restrooms, and cafeterias.

  Regular disinfection of surfaces can help reduce the risk of virus transmission.

- Flexible Attendance Policies:

 To encourage students and staff to stay home when they are sick, schools should consider implementing flexible attendance policies.

 This may include allowing for remote learning options or not penalizing students for absences related to illness.

Guidelines for Parents and Teachers

Parents and teachers play a critical role in preventing the spread of Parvovirus B19 in schools.

By following these guidelines, they can help protect students and the broader community:

- Monitoring Symptoms: Parents should monitor their children for symptoms of Parvovirus B19, particularly during times of increased community transmission.

 Teachers should also be vigilant in observing students for signs of illness.

- Keeping Sick Children at Home: Children who exhibit symptoms of Parvovirus B19, such as fever, rash, or joint pain, should be kept home from school until they are no longer contagious.

 This is particularly important during the early stages of the illness when the virus is most likely to spread.

- Encouraging Hygiene Practices: Both parents and teachers should reinforce the importance of good hygiene practices, such as regular handwashing, covering coughs and sneezes, and avoiding close contact with sick individuals.

- Communicating with the School: Parents should inform the school if their child has been diagnosed with Parvovirus B19, so that appropriate measures can be taken to prevent further spread. Teachers should also report any suspected cases to school administrators promptly.

The Role of Remote Learning as a Contingency

In the event of a significant Parvovirus B19 outbreak, remote learning may become a necessary contingency to prevent further transmission and protect vulnerable students and staff.

- Preparing for Remote Learning: Schools should ensure that they have the infrastructure and resources in place to switch to remote learning if needed.

 This includes providing access to online learning platforms, ensuring students have the necessary devices and internet access, and offering training to teachers on how to deliver effective remote instruction.

- Communication with Parents: Clear communication with parents about the conditions under which remote learning would be implemented and how it would be managed is essential.

 Schools should provide guidelines on how parents can support their children's learning at home and maintain a structured learning environment.

- Supporting Students with Special Needs: Schools should have plans in place to support students with special needs during remote learning, including providing appropriate accommodations and resources to ensure these students can continue their education with minimal disruption.

Case Studies from Previous Outbreaks

Looking at past Parvovirus B19 outbreaks can provide valuable insights into how schools can effectively manage such situations.

Here are a few key lessons from previous cases:

- Early Identification and Isolation: In schools that successfully managed outbreaks, early identification of cases and prompt isolation of affected individuals were crucial in preventing widespread transmission.

 This underscores the importance of training staff to recognize symptoms and take swift action.

- Collaboration with Health Authorities: Effective collaboration with local health departments was another common factor in successful outbreak management.

 Schools that worked closely with health officials to implement control measures and communicate with the community were better able to contain the virus.

- Flexibility and Adaptation: Schools that demonstrated flexibility in their response—such as by adjusting attendance policies, offering remote learning, and modifying schedules—were able to minimize disruption to education while protecting the health of students and staff.

By learning from these examples, schools can better prepare for the potential impact of Parvovirus B19 on the new school year and take proactive steps to protect their communities.

5. Steps to Take If Infected

Recognizing the Symptoms Early

Early recognition of Parvovirus B19 infection is key to managing the disease and preventing its spread.

Individuals should be aware of the following symptoms and take appropriate action if they develop:

- Initial Symptoms: The early signs of infection can be nonspecific and may include mild fever, fatigue, and respiratory symptoms such as a sore throat or runny nose. These symptoms often precede the appearance of the rash by several days.

- Facial Rash: The characteristic "slapped cheek" rash is a hallmark of Parvovirus B19 infection. It typically appears suddenly and is bright red in color, affecting both cheeks symmetrically.

- Lacy Body Rash: A few days after the facial rash, a lacy or reticular rash may develop on the trunk and limbs. This rash can be mildly itchy and may come and go over several days.

- Joint Pain: In some cases, particularly in older children and adults, joint pain and swelling may occur. This symptom can affect the hands, wrists, knees, and ankles, and may persist for weeks.

Treatment Options and Home Care

 There is no specific antiviral treatment for Parvovirus B19, so management focuses on relieving symptoms and supporting recovery. Most cases can be managed at home with the following measures:

- Rest: Rest is important to help the body recover from the infection. Children and adults with Parvovirus B19 should be encouraged to take it easy and avoid strenuous activities until they feel better.

- Hydration: Staying well-hydrated is essential, especially if fever is present. Drinking plenty of fluids such as water, clear broths, and oral rehydration solutions can help prevent dehydration.

- Fever and Pain Management: Over-the-counter medications such as acetaminophen or ibuprofen can be used to reduce fever and relieve joint pain. Aspirin should be avoided in children due to the risk of Reye's syndrome, a rare but serious condition.

- Skin Care: The rash associated with Parvovirus B19 can be itchy. Applying calamine lotion or a cool compress to the affected areas can help soothe the skin and reduce discomfort.

- Avoiding Triggers: The body rash may be exacerbated by heat, sunlight, or stress. Individuals with the rash should try to avoid these triggers to prevent worsening of symptoms.

When to Seek Medical Attention

 While most cases of Parvovirus B19 are mild and resolve on their own, there are situations where medical attention is necessary:

- Severe Anemia: Individuals with underlying blood disorders, such as sickle cell disease or hereditary spherocytosis, who develop symptoms of severe anemia—such as extreme fatigue, shortness of breath, or paleness—should seek medical care immediately.

- Pregnancy: Pregnant women who are exposed to Parvovirus B19 or develop symptoms should contact their healthcare provider promptly, as the infection can pose serious risks to the fetus.

- Immunocompromised Individuals: Those with weakened immune systems who develop symptoms of Parvovirus B19 should seek medical attention, as they may be at risk for chronic infection or severe complications.

- Prolonged or Severe Symptoms: If symptoms persist for more than a few weeks, or if the individual experiences severe joint pain, swelling, or other concerning symptoms, a healthcare provider should be consulted.

Coping with the Psychological Impact

 Dealing with a Parvovirus B19 infection, particularly for pregnant women or those with underlying health conditions, can be stressful. Coping strategies may include:

- Seeking Support: Talking to friends, family, or a counselor can help individuals cope with the anxiety and uncertainty associated with the illness.

- Staying Informed: Understanding the nature of the virus and the typical course of the disease can help alleviate fears and misconceptions.

- Managing Stress: Engaging in stress-reducing activities such as meditation, deep breathing exercises, or gentle physical activity can help improve overall well-being during recovery.

Recovery Process and Returning to School

The recovery process from Parvovirus B19 varies depending on the severity of the infection and the individual's overall health.

Most people recover fully within a few weeks, but joint pain and fatigue can linger in some cases.

- Gradual Return to Activities: After the acute phase of the illness, individuals should gradually return to their normal activities. Children returning to school should do so only when they feel well enough and are no longer contagious.

- Follow-up Care: In cases where complications arise, such as severe anemia or chronic joint pain, follow-up care with a healthcare provider may be necessary to monitor recovery and manage ongoing symptoms.

- Preventing Recurrence: While reinfection with Parvovirus B19 is rare due to lasting immunity, individuals should continue to practice good hygiene and take preventive measures to avoid other infections.

 Taking these steps can help manage the infection effectively and support a smooth recovery, minimizing the impact on the individual's health and daily life.

6. Community and Government Response

Public Health Policies

Effective public health policies are crucial in controlling the spread of Parvovirus B19 and managing outbreaks when they occur.

These policies should focus on prevention, early detection, and rapid response:

- Surveillance Systems: Public health authorities should maintain robust surveillance systems to monitor the incidence of Parvovirus B19 in the community.

 This includes tracking cases in schools, daycare centers, and healthcare facilities.

- Reporting and Communication: Clear guidelines should be established for reporting cases of Parvovirus B19 to public health authorities.

 Timely communication between schools, healthcare providers, and public health officials is essential for coordinating an effective response.

- Guidance for Schools: Public health agencies should provide schools with guidelines on how to prevent and manage outbreaks of Parvovirus B19.

 This includes recommendations for hygiene practices, case identification, and isolation protocols.

- Outreach to Vulnerable Populations: Special attention should be given to protecting vulnerable populations, such as pregnant women, immunocompromised individuals, and those with chronic health conditions.

 Public health campaigns should target these groups with information on how to reduce their risk of infection.

Role of Schools in Public Health Initiatives

 Schools play a vital role in public health initiatives aimed at controlling the spread of Parvovirus B19.

 By partnering with public health authorities, schools can contribute to the overall health and safety of the community:

- Implementing Preventive Measures: Schools should adopt preventive measures, such as promoting hand hygiene, ensuring proper cleaning and disinfection, and educating students and staff about the virus.

- Collaborating with Health Authorities: Schools should work closely with local health departments to monitor the health of students and staff, report cases of illness, and implement control measures during outbreaks.

- Providing Health Education: Schools should incorporate health education into the curriculum, teaching students about the importance of hygiene, the symptoms of common illnesses like Parvovirus B19, and how to prevent the spread of infections.
- Supporting Vaccination Programs: While there is no vaccine for Parvovirus B19, schools can support vaccination programs for other preventable diseases, which can help reduce the overall burden of illness and make it easier to manage outbreaks.

Collaboration with Health Authorities

 Collaboration between schools, healthcare providers, and public health authorities is essential for managing Parvovirus B19 outbreaks and protecting public health:
- Coordinated Response: Schools and health authorities should develop coordinated response plans for Parvovirus B19 outbreaks. This includes establishing communication channels, sharing data on cases, and working together to implement control measures.

- Community Education: Health authorities should work with schools to educate the community about Parvovirus B19, including how it spreads, how to recognize symptoms, and what to do if an infection is suspected.

- Providing Resources: Public health agencies should provide schools with resources, such as educational materials, hygiene supplies, and guidance on managing outbreaks, to help them effectively respond to Parvovirus B19.

Awareness Campaigns and Educational Programs

 Raising awareness about Parvovirus B19 through public health campaigns and educational programs is key to preventing the spread of the virus and protecting vulnerable populations:

- Public Awareness Campaigns: Public health authorities should launch awareness campaigns that inform the public about Parvovirus B19, its symptoms, and how to prevent infection. These campaigns should target both the general public and specific at-risk groups.
- School-Based Education Programs: Schools should implement educational programs that teach students about hygiene practices, the importance of staying home when sick, and how to protect themselves and others from infectious diseases.

- Community Engagement: Engaging community leaders, parents, and local organizations in awareness campaigns can help amplify the message and encourage widespread adoption of preventive measures.

 Through a coordinated effort involving public health policies, school initiatives, and community engagement, the spread of Parvovirus B19 can be effectively controlled, minimizing its impact on public health and the new school year.

7. Conclusion

Recap of Key Points

Parvovirus B19, commonly known as "slapped cheek disease," is a highly contagious virus that primarily affects children but can have serious consequences for pregnant women, immunocompromised individuals, and those with underlying health conditions. The virus spreads easily in community settings such as schools, where close contact among students facilitates transmission.

Preventing the spread of Parvovirus B19 requires a multifaceted approach that includes good hygiene practices, early recognition of symptoms, and timely intervention during outbreaks.

Schools play a critical role in implementing preventive measures and collaborating with public health authorities to manage the virus's impact on the school community.

Importance of Preparedness and Prevention

Preparedness is key to minimizing the impact of Parvovirus B19 on the new school year. Schools, parents, and public health authorities must work together to implement preventive measures, educate the community, and respond effectively to outbreaks.

By taking proactive steps, the spread of the virus can be controlled, protecting the health of students, staff, and the broader community.

Final Thoughts on Protecting the School Community

 As the new school year begins, the threat of Parvovirus B19 serves as a reminder of the importance of vigilance and preparedness in managing infectious diseases.

 By staying informed, practicing good hygiene, and working together, we can ensure that schools remain safe and healthy environments for all students and staff.

Please use the next few pages
for your notes and debates.